The Healthy Family Handbook

The Healthy Family Handbook

Creating Physical & Emotional Nutrition at Home

Andrea Frank Henkart

Photographs by Reggie Henkart

Foreword by Becky Natrajan, M.D.

Family Freedom, Inc.

Marin County, CA

The Healthy Family Handbook

Cover/Book Design & Layout: Charis Santillie, CAS Designs, www.cas-designs.com

Family Freedom, Inc.
P.O. Box 5494
Novato, CA 94948
www.coolcommunication.com

ISBN 0-9720738-1-7

Second Edition
Printed in the United States of America

A Note to Readers

No liability is assumed with respect to the use of information herein. The contents in this book are the opinion of the author and contributors and may not represent the consensus of opinion of the medical profession at this time. The contents of this book are not intended to be used to treat, cure, mitigate or diagnose any medical condition. As with any health program, readers are advised to consult with a physician before making any changes that could affect their health.

Contents

Acknowledgments

I offer my appreciation and gratitude to John and Cher Anderson and Jim and Kathy Coover for creating the #1 health and wellness products in America and beyond. A company is only as good as the people who run it and Isagenix™ International is OUTSTANDING!

Ron Reid and Linda Upham deserve loving thanks for their patient leadership and spectacular team support. They are extraordinary friends who bring true meaning to "Isagenix Family."

Special thanks to my contributors, friends and colleagues for your assistance, collaboration and suggestions: Ellen Bradley and Paul Ganus, Dr. George Boris, John and Janet Burton, Jack Canfield, Kathy Coover, Tony and Randi Escobar, Dr. Dennis Harper, Kathy and Todd Humphreys, Dr. Tom McNeilis, Beth Miller, Dr. Becky Natrajan and Dan Maes, Lissa Rovetch, Charis Santillie, Jimmy Smith, my editor Mark Steisel, Marilyn

Territo, Dr. Cynthia M. Watson and Dr. Jay Williams.

My loving thanks go to the most talented, award-winning photographer in the world, my husband Reggie. I also want to thank my son, Quest, for excellent advice and input. And to my daughter, Journey, thank you for your continuous support, partnership and editing skills.

Last, but certainly not least, I offer my special thanks to my dear friends, John and Bonnie Gray for introducing my family to the wonderful world of Isagenix.

Foreword

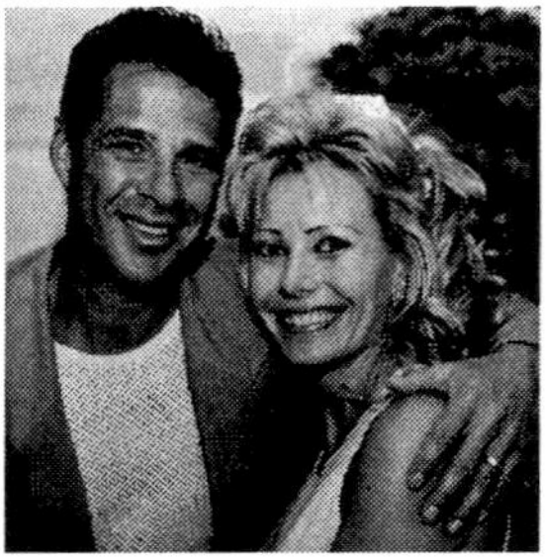

I am a practicing Gastroenterologist in Tucson, Arizona and have been in practice for eleven years. My husband, Dan Maes, has been in the nutrition industry for twelve years. Together, we have witnessed thousands of lives change through good nutritional supplementation, exercise and a balanced diet. We have made it our life's mission to educate people on the importance of nutritional replenishment and the essential need to cleanse our bodies of accumulated dangerous, often deadly toxins.

We are being bombarded with toxins twenty-four hours a day in the form of air, water and ground pollution. There are so many pesticides and insecticides on our fruits and vegetables that pesticides seem to have become a part of the food chain. Animals raised for consumption are injected with hormones, steroids and antibiotics. These toxins have a serious detrimental effect on our vital organs and immune systems.

America is in a true health crisis. 44 million people suffer from arthritis, 18 million have diabetes, 17 million suffer from asthma, 1 in 8 develop breast cancer and 18 million children are obese. 81% of our nation is overweight. Last year in this country alone, over 2.8 billion prescriptions were prescribed! Children are facing twin epidemics in this country: Obesity and Type-II Diabetes. There are also an exorbitant number of children being diagnosed with "brain chemistry issues," such as ADD and ADHD.

Because our soils have become so depleted, many of us are minerally depleted and in many cases, minerally bankrupt. Minerals are essential for 90% of our bodily functions. You cannot absorb vitamins if your body does not have the necessary minerals it needs.

Good nutrition can help prevent many of the health-related problems facing us today, yet we continue to make poor nutritional choices for our children and ourselves. Our kids continue to eat massive amounts of junk food, which is deplete of vital amino acids and proteins. It does not provide the essential building blocks necessary for developing strong brains, bones and immune systems.

Health and Wellness is a family affair. In my professional opinion, if you don't take care of yourself and your family now, it is not a matter of "if you are going to get sick," it is just a matter of "when." When you take an active role in keeping your body internally strong, you send a powerful message to your kids. You demonstrate that it is cool to be healthy. When the entire family is nutritionally on track, the family unit becomes stronger on all levels.

Fifteen months ago, my family and I were introduced to a comprehensive nutritional system that changed our lives. John Anderson, a genius formulator in Chandler, Arizona, created a nutritional cleansing system that provides the brain and body with 242 essential nutrients, gentle pure cleansing herbs, high-grade whey protein, amino acids and 70 organic, ionic plant minerals.

Isagenix, which means "Balanced Life" in Latin, has a special digestive delivery system that allows the body to absorb all these essential nutrients. Combined with exercise and a balanced diet, this nutritional system can help your family avoid future obesity, disease and illness.

Health and wellness is a major focus in my own household and Isagenix has become a critical part of our lifestyle. Sometimes my children attend our educational and nutritional seminars. We are very open with our children about how toxins in our environment can adversely affect our health. My son knows more about cellular cleansing than most adults!

It has become a family ritual to have an Isagenix shake every morning so we can start our day with excellent brain chemistry and clarity of thought. If America were to join us on this mission, I absolutely believe that everyone would face fewer health challenges.

The Healthy Family Handbook addresses the issues that challenge families on a daily basis. I love Andrea's message because it provides a strong foundation for a healthy home life. I had the pleasure of spending time with Andrea and her family. Her commitment to her own children is the key to her ability to pass on such an important message.

I sincerely hope *The Healthy Family Handbook* inspires you and your family to incorporate safe, effective cleansing and nutritional replenishment, along with valuable communication skills for a lifetime of optimum health, wellness and renewed spirit.

Becky Natrajan, MD
Gastroenterologist
Tucson, AZ

WHAT MATTERS

(Author unknown)

One hundred years from now,
It will not matter what kind of car I drove,
What kind of house I lived in,
How much I had in my bank account,
Nor what my clothes looked like.
But the world may be a little better because
I was important in the life of a child.

Create Health & Harmony at Home

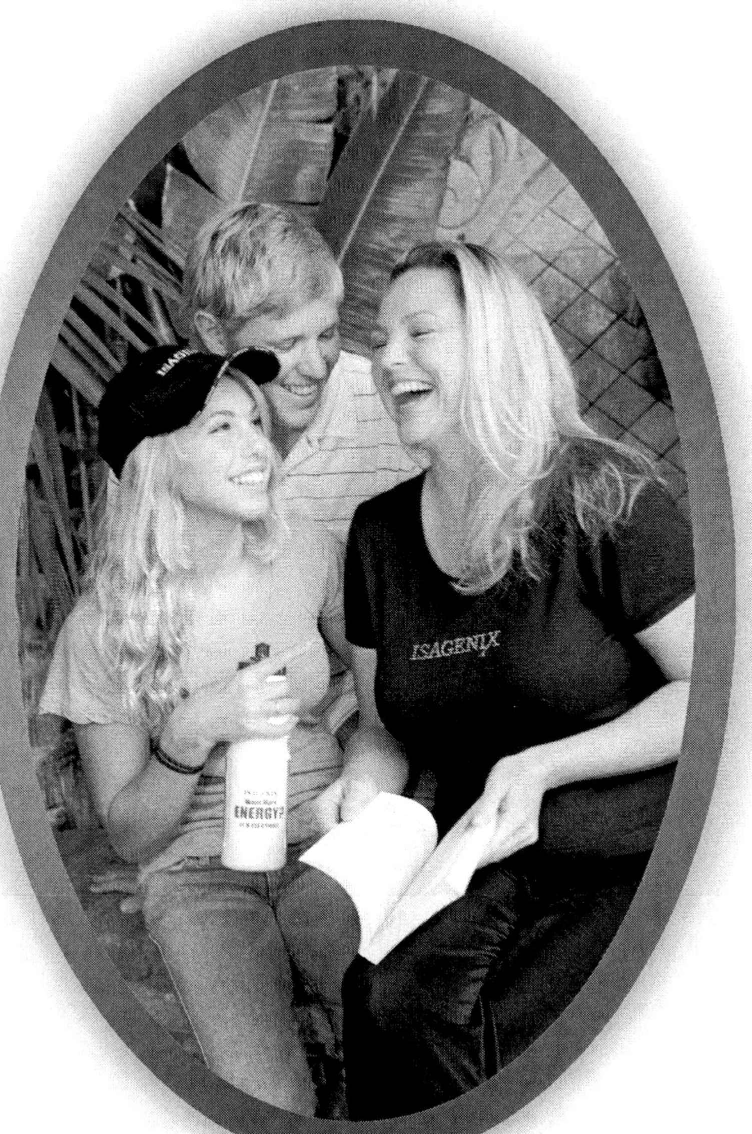

Chapter 1

Create Health & Harmony at Home

"Imagine the joy of learning to connect with your son or daughter on a level that overcomes all the petty conflicts. Andrea and her daughter, Journey, have figured out a way to not only get along, but also to celebrate each other's spirit."

Oprah Winfrey

Balancing family life and work has become more hectic than ever. With our to-do-lists in hand and cell phones attached to our ears, we speed through the day with such urgency that we become irritated with the slightest setback. Children seem to suffer the most from our exceedingly permissive and fast-paced world.

A rapidly increasing number of kids are overweight, over-stressed and over medicated. Children between the ages of one to seventeen account for seven percent of all antidepressant prescriptions. Attention Deficit Disorder (ADD), Attention Deficit/

Hyperactive Disorder (ADHD), adolescent drinking, teen suicide and school shootings are at an all time high.

To make matters worse, we are in an obesity epidemic that is filtering down to the playpen. According to the American Heart Association, more than ten percent of American children between the ages of two and five are overweight. Pediatricians and gastroenterologists continue to link this obesity epidemic to an increasing number of children with diabetes, high blood pressure and liver disease. Experts blame the prevalence of junk food marketed to kids, too much television, not enough exercise, and the decline in the number of families who take the time to sit down and eat together.

The explosion in obesity rates and disease has made us all keenly aware of the need to make changes in our collective behavior. When it comes to our kids, we must make sure the message is about healthful living, not just weight. In all eagerness to stem the obesity epidemic, parents must make sure they do not damage their kids' self esteem by reinforcing negative body images. It is rare to find an adolescent girl who feels good about her body; boys are increasingly affected as well. It can be difficult to change negative body esteem and eating habits once they have been established.

The media feeds into this frenzy by suggesting that looking a certain way can get you what you want out of life. With all the nipping, tucking and lifting shown on TV, it is no wonder that girls are uncomfortable and untrusting of their own bodies, while boys turn to steroids and other methods to alter the way they look. Instead of buying into the media's approach, I highly recommend that parents change the focus from looking good to being healthy.

In my professional opinion, we have become too permissive as a culture. Parents are too busy, some are afraid to say "No" to their kids, while others just don't know what to do. I have met parents who give up, ignore inappropriate behavior, or pull in the reins and become overly strict. Authoritative parenting can be just as detrimental as over-permissive parenting. It is vital that we create balance in our families so our children can grow up with a strong sense of respect for themselves and the world around them.

Tradition has it that parents know best, yet most of us are thrust into the role of parenting without any previous training. Parents often rely on yesterday's solutions to solve today's problems. Sometimes it is difficult to know the best parenting approach to use with our children; after all, kids do not come with an instruction manual. If they did, teenagers would confuse matters by changing the manual daily!

Using cool communication techniques and proven success strategies, my daughter, Journey, and I have inspired thousands of parents and kids around the world to talk to, and even understand each other. In our workshops, keynote speeches and books, we provide families with a much-needed perspective from both the parents' and kids' sides in understanding this often turbulent and frustrating relationship.

Our work has been highly influenced by our dear friend of 20 years, John Gray, Ph.D., author of the bestselling book, *Men Are From Mars, Women Are From Venus*. That is why my interest peaked one day when John approached me and told me about a relatively new company he was involved in called, Isagenix™. He said, "The vitamins, protein shake, cleanse drink and minerals changed my life. It works so effectively for everyone because it helps to balance brain chemistry. This naturally lowers stress levels and when that occurs, you experience fat-burning, appetite control and a sense of well-being."

Researchers have identified that a diet rich in nutrients, vitamins and amino acids may enhance brain function as well as improve cognitive abilities, concentration, vision and nervous system function. Based on this information and trusting John and knowing the depth of his integrity, I tried the products. Then I got my husband and two children to try them. We unanimously agreed that this was a fabulous way to improve our lifestyle from a health and wellness perspective.

A New Way of Living

When Master Formulator, John Anderson, founder and CEO of Isagenix International, introduced the Isagenix IsaKids™ nutritional program at the second annual Isagenix convention, the excitement in the room was soaring. I heard parents exclaim:

- "Finally, something to balance my kids out."
- "Maybe this will help the problems we have in our family."
- "If I get my son on the products, maybe he'll behave better."
- "Good nutrition for my children. Just what I've been waiting for."

I felt compelled to let parents know that good nutrition is only a piece of the parenting pie. Eating well, exercising and using the best vitamins available are invaluable to your family's overall health. However, if you and your kids do not have a healthy relationship enhanced with successful communication skills, you may not have the complete results you are hoping for.

I wrote *The Healthy Family Handbook* to provide you with simple, easy-to-follow tools to create health and harmony at home. My hope is that you will use the techniques in this book to develop and maintain positive relationships with your children through all the various phases and stages of development.

I am an author and international motivational speaker, specializing in communication skills and life balance for the family. I studied basic nutrition and became a Holistic Health Counselor in 1980. I am not a practicing nutritionist, but because I believe so strongly in the Isagenix Nutritional System™ and have experienced incredible results first hand, I felt it was vitally important to weave Isagenix product information throughout this book to create a link between positive parenting and healthy nutrition.

My contributing writers from the Isagenix Medical Advisory Board, George Boris, M.D.,

Dennis Harper, M.D., Tom McNeilis, M.D., Becky Natrajan, M.D. and Cynthia M. Watson, M.D., along with experts Tony Escobar and Marilyn Territo, further explain the details of healthy living and its effects on the family. Their work solidifies the link between physical and emotional nutrition and allows families to begin to make a difference in the way they choose to parent.

I encourage you to combine the Isagenix Nutritional System with effective communication and lots of love to create a winning recipe that will sustain and enrich you and your children for years to come.

Thank you for joining me on this path of awareness and thank you for taking the time to be outstanding parents.

> ***Let's not only catch our children being successful, let's set them up for success.***
>
> *Eugene Anderson, Ed.D.*

Inspire Your Kids with Healthy Nutrition

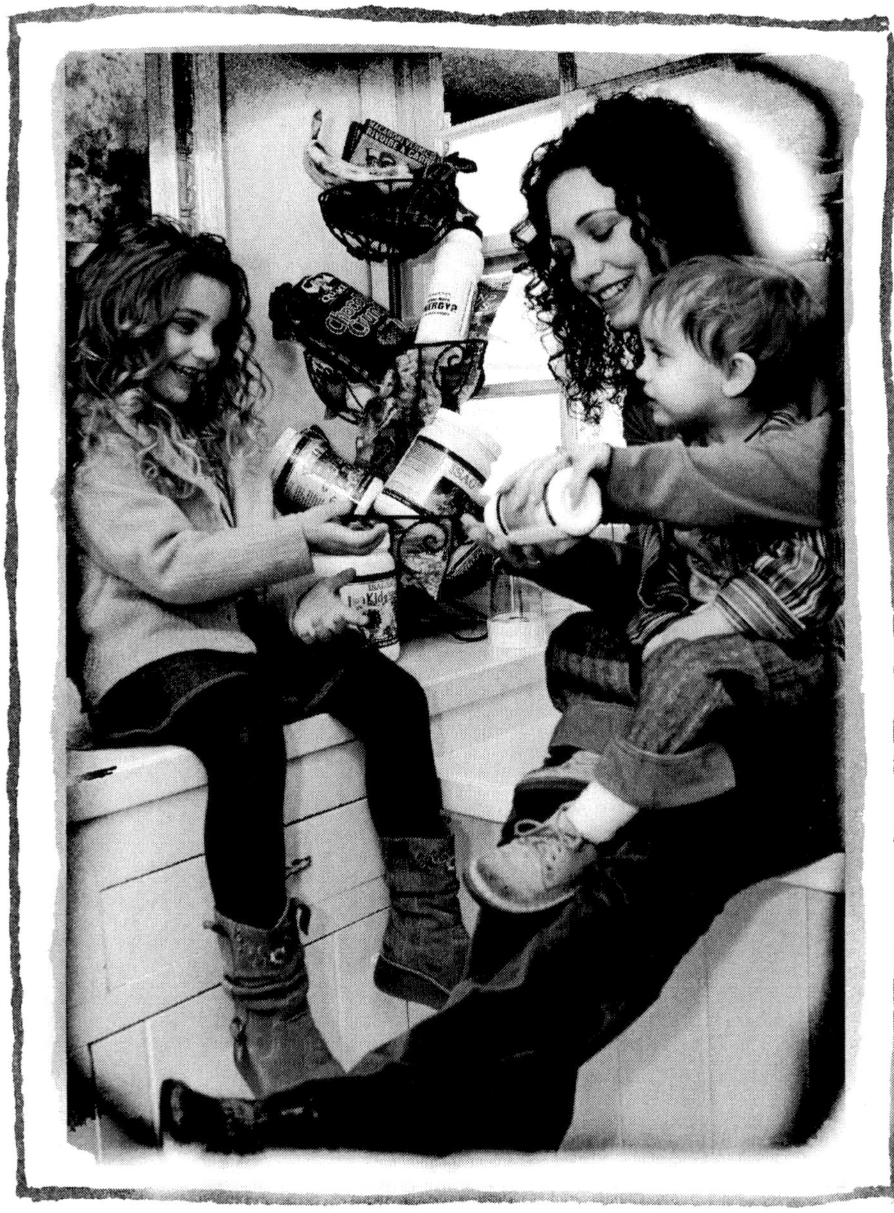

Chapter 2

Inspire Your Kids with Healthy Nutrition

Getting kids to eat healthy meals can be a nightmare. In a world filled with junk food and unrelenting advertisements, it is difficult to make sure your kids are getting the proper nutrients they need. Parents often wonder:

- Are my kids eating the right foods?
- Are they getting enough protein?
- How can I get them to eat more fruits and vegetables?
- Will they ever eat anything other than peanut butter sandwiches and French fries?

Statistics show that soda, French fries, potato chips, hamburgers and chocolate comprise 70% of the American diet. No wonder America's health is so awful! Unfortunately, countries around the world are quickly catching up. Diets rich in fresh fruits and vegetables have given way to processed foods filled with fat, salt and sugar. New estimates indicate that about half a million children in Europe are combating the same kinds of health problems suffered by middle-aged adults, simply because they weigh too much.

Most experts agree that breakfast is the most important meal of the day. Kids who skip breakfast or eat unhealthy sugary foods, such as cereal or pastries, may have difficulty concentrating. Studies continue to show that ADD/ADHD may be caused or exacerbated by poor nutrition. According to an article in The New England Journal of Medicine, a diet composed of largely saturated fat, animal fatty acids, cholesterol and trans-fatty acids may increase the risk of diabetes, heart-disease and cancer. To improve your family's health, serve unprocessed, natural and organic foods as often as you can. The more life in your food, the more life it will give you.

Parents Can Finally Relax

Isagenix has a program for children that makes nutrition delicious, easy and fun. Kids who follow the Isagenix program and eat a healthy, well-balanced diet receive the precise nutrients they need to build strong, healthy bodies.

A daily IsaKids™ Super Shake is the perfect way to ensure that your children get the essential proteins and amino acids needed to boost their brain chemistry and support their growing bodies and minds. The IsaKids shake contains 17 grams of low-lactose, hormone-free, organic whey protein from New Zealand, naturally occurring amino acids, an enzyme delivery system for assimilation and organic ionic and trace minerals. Your kids can also enjoy the Chocolate and French Vanilla Isagenix IsaLean™ Shakes that you use every day.

Whey protein is not new; it has been available for hundreds of years. It is a high quality, complete protein that contains all of the essential amino acids required by the body each and every day. Whey protein provides energy to the body and a boost to the immune system. Athletes have also used whey protein after strenuous activity to help repair their bodies and rebuild muscle tissue.

Dr. Bryan Turner, of the Jordan Health and Wellness Center in South Jordan, Utah says, "The organic whey protein in the Isagenix IsaLean™ Shake is an excellent source of the nutritional building blocks necessary for our bodies to maximize glutathione production. Glutathione, (pronounced glue-ta-thigh-on) is an important molecule that works inside cells to defeat free radicals. Free radicals damage enzymes and the DNA, which leads to physical changes associated with aging and disease. With consistent use of the shakes, one would expect powerful anti-aging effects."

According to an online Isagenix newsletter, scientists in Denmark found that subjects who took whey protein every day experienced a significant drop in the hormones that produce stress and a forty-eight percent increase in tryptophan levels. Tryptophan is an amino acid that your brain uses to make serotonin, which gives you a sense of well-being. Additional studies found that whey immediately boosts mental alertness by fifteen percent. Doctors and health professionals all over America are encouraging families to add the Isagenix shake into their diet on a daily basis to increase energy, stamina and overall health.

Making the Transition

When you introduce new foods or supplements to your kids, don't nag or lecture them. If they feel pressured or forced into trying something new, your picky eaters may get pickier. Forcing your kids to finish everything on their plates can cause them to overeat, rebel or stop eating altogether as they attempt to maintain a sense of control over their lives. Chances are that nagging them will create unnecessary power struggles.

To start your children on a lifetime of eating nutritiously, practice what you preach. Add healthy eating habits to your lifestyle and follow the Isagenix program to cleanse, rejuvenate and revitalize your system.

- Have a delicious, nourishing Isagenix Shake every morning with your children.
- Eat fruits and vegetables in front of your kids.
- Eliminate as much junk food from the family diet as possible.
- Take your vitamins and antioxidants with your kids; make it a family routine.
- Be sure that you and your children drink plenty of water rather than soda and empty calorie fruit drinks.
- Establish healthy routines early and stick to them.

Cookies, candy and soda can lead to a sugar path of no return, so provide a better alternative by keeping Isagenix Slim Cakes™ in your pantry. Each delicious cookie has less than 190 calories. This tasty treat is loaded with vitamins and minerals and contains nine grams of fiber, five grams of flax seed and five grams of protein. Put a couple of Slim Cakes in your children's lunch box so they can share them with their friends.

Kids also love the Isagenix IsaLean™ Bars, which are a great tasting meal alternative or snack. Available in two flavors: Chocolate Dipped Honey Peanut and Yogurt Dipped Oatmeal Raisin, each Kosher certified bar has 17 grams of natural protein, 32-34 grams of carbohydrates, 2 grams of fiber, 250 calories, lots of trace minerals and no trans-fats. Freeze an IsaLean Bar, then take it to school or sports games for a "cool" treat.

Get Them Involved

Another way to get your children interested in nutritious food is to let them help you prepare meals. Little kids feel proud when they can lend a hand, especially when you give them credit and express your appreciation. Teach your kids to make their own nourishing IsaLean shakes. You will find a variety of kid-friendly recipes in the back of this book.

As your children grow, involve them in meal planning and shopping, as well as preparation. If your teenagers don't like what you cook, don't take it personally. Keep your kitchen stocked with fresh fruit, vegetables and nutritious items so they can prepare food and snacks for themselves. When your kids observe you eating wholesome meals and avoiding junk food, they may follow your lead and automatically reach for something healthy like IsaLean™ Creamy Chicken Soup.

This savory, hot soup is fortified with the same nutritious profile of vitamins and enzymes as the IsaLean shake, including IsaLyte™ trace mineral citrate, the best organic whey protein, and naturally occurring amino acids. It has 18.5 grams of protein, 4 grams of fiber and only 3 grams of sugar derived from honey. A delicious, healthy and complete meal alternative, there simply is no better way to provide the maximum amount of nutrients in the fewest number of calories.

IsaLean™ Soup is designed to be used synergistically with the Isagenix System. You can also use it as a meal supplement or after-school snack. It is easy if you are in a hurry;

simply add two scoops of soup to 8-12 ounces of hot water and let it steep for approximately two minutes—you don't even need a microwave!

If your kids are not eating enough fruits and vegetables, let them drink their fruit! Isagenix™ IsaFruits is a wonderful alternative to sugary drinks. Flavonoid-rich berries shield you and your family from invading free radicals that can cause disease. Red tomato and pomegranate lycopene coupled with carrot and papaya beta-carotene fortify healthy body structures, like eyes, skin, lungs, colon, liver, and the prostate in men. Acerola and cherries supply Vitamin C. Pineapple and noni adaptogens, and cranberry tannins serve as a buffer for your immune system. A blend of digestive enzymes ensures maximum absorption, and probiotic bacteria helps the body maintain a proper balance of intestinal flora. Apple pectin, oat bran, rice bran and flaxseed form a smooth, hearty texture and supply fiber and essential fatty acids.

Just one small scoop of Isagenix™ IsaFruits mixed with water is a quick and delicious way to get the benefits of eating a variety of antioxidant-packed whole fruits daily. Kids love the taste of Isagenix™ IsaFruits and teenagers love how easy it is to make! Add fresh, organic fruit and ice to make your own smoothie. It is perfect for your life-on-the-go.

We have all heard that we should drink eight to ten glasses of water a day to maintain hydration. Even a small degree of dehydration can lead to a reduction in both mental and physical performance. Water is one of the most important essential nutrients for children, so keep your family hydrated. It regulates body temperature, transports nutrients and oxygen to the blood, removes waste, lubricates joints and protects organs and tissues in the body. Pack a bottle of water in your child's lunch instead of soda or juice and don't forget to carry a bottle with you when you go out for the day.

Numerous studies have shown that when you provide your children with wholesome food, they continue to crave good nutrition for the rest of their lives. They take their cues from the adults around them and learn by imitation and identification as well as discussion. It is never too late to start demonstrating good habits. Your kids will learn valuable skills and develop nutritional habits that will last a lifetime.

Mankind owes to the child
the best it has to give.

U.N. Declaration

Practice What You Preach

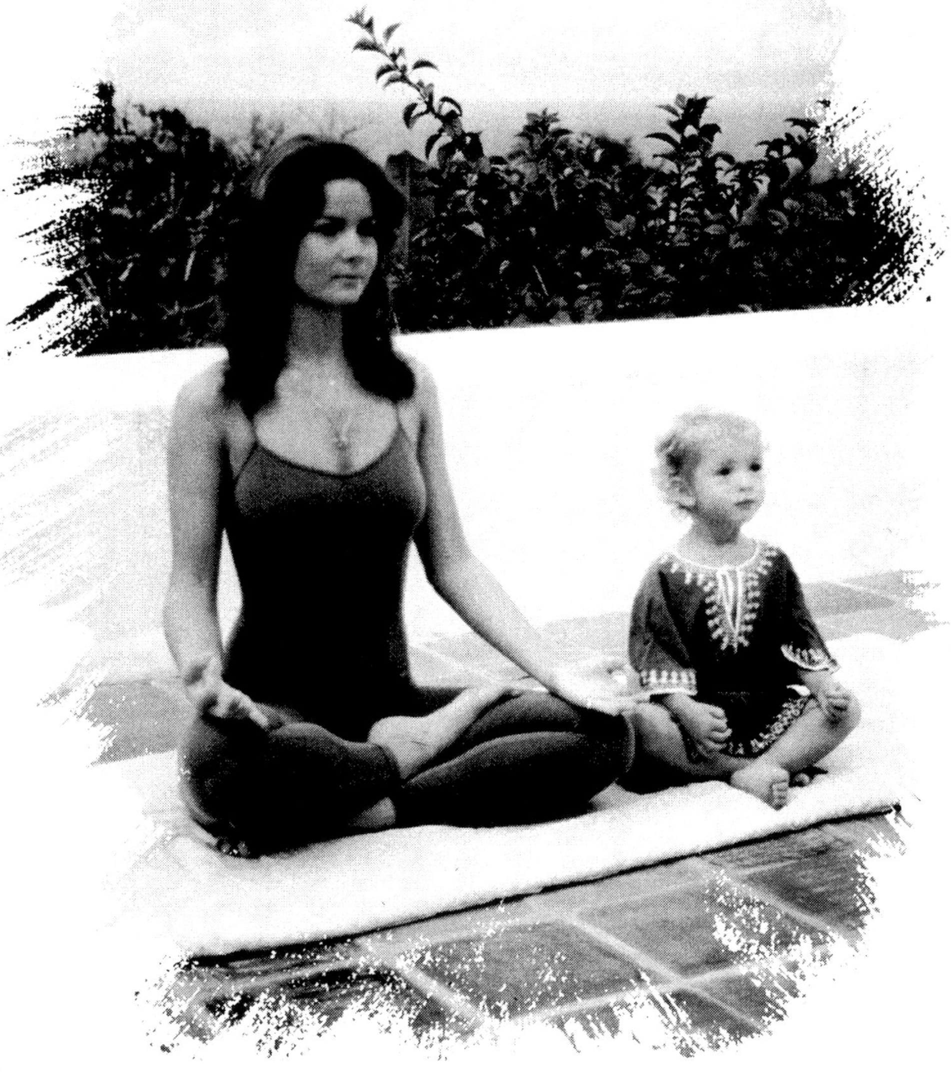

Chapter 3

Practice What You Preach

The art of parenting takes a little bit of wisdom and a great deal of patience. Kids today are bombarded by negative and often conflicting influences from their peers and the pressures of society. Your children depend on you to provide stability and guidance.

Embody the values you want your children to possess. Are you honest? Are you reliable? Do you swear? Do you drive fast? Do you gossip about your friends or family members? While you may think these actions are relatively harmless, your children are always watching, learning and mimicking your behavior. In their minds, your actions give them license for similar conduct. We all know there is no such thing as a perfect family, but it is up to us to do the best we can to set an outstanding example.

Not only do your kids watch how you behave, they also listen to what you say and how you say it. If you are overweight or have no energy, the last thing you want is someone telling you how fat and lazy you are. Insulting or chastising can undermine their confidence and self-esteem. Negative talk does not inspire kids; it exasperates and discourages them.

Give your children enough breathing space so they can come up with creative ideas to solve problems on their own. Think before you speak. Demonstrate good communication skills by talking to your kids the way you would want someone to talk to you if you were in the same situation.

The most meaningful lessons that you can teach are delivered in clear examples of the way you live your life. When conflicts arise, talk about the steps you are taking to resolve them so your kids can learn how to problem solve. Encourage your kids to confront their feelings and express their full range of emotions instead of running away from them. Family therapy, personal growth seminars and books on parenting can be instrumental in helping you to acquire coping skills to confront and work through uncomfortable feelings.

When your kids do express their feelings, be prepared for everything from sulking to door slamming. Don't take it personally. Instead of getting angry and giving up, help them find positive ways to express their changing thoughts and negative behavior.

- Let your kids talk on the phone with friends so they can share their innermost feelings.

- Give your son or daughter a punching bag or pillow to safely let out aggressive behavior.

- Read with them to open their minds to the infinite possibilities of life.

- Encourage your kids to take part in community service so they can learn the rewards of giving to others, instead of constantly dwelling on themselves.

Think about the type of examples you set for your children. School-aged kids can be cruel and teenagers can be disrespectful, but remember that babies are not born mean or rude. Kids learn behavior from their circle of influence: family, friends, school and the media.

Model the Behavior You Expect

Be aware of what you say about your family, your neighbors or the people around you. Are you quick to judge others? Are you overly harsh? How well do you take care of yourself? It is difficult to convince a kid to calm down and stop screaming if you are always stressed out and yelling. Be aware of the powerful influence you have on your children and the lessons you are teaching them through your words and actions.

To be a healthy influence, keep yourself at your optimum level of health and vitality. Get rid of the toxins that have accumulated in your system. Set down that can of diet soda, put out that cigarette and cleanse your body from the inside out.

Why do we need to cleanse internally? According to Dr. Becky Natrajan, "We are nutritionally bankrupt!" She points out that:

- There are seventy-two pesticides and insecticides in our fruits and vegetables.
- Industrial dumping is continually being poured into our ground.
- Our drinking water is full of heavy metals and bacteria.
- We breathe air full of fumes and pollution.
- Our soils are depleted.

The results are frightening! Last year:

- There were 1.1 million deaths from heart disease.
- 18 million were diagnosed with Type-II Diabetes.
- 770 thousand people died from cancer.

- 1 out of 7 pregnancies ended in miscarriage.
- 85% of these cases did not have a genetic history.

The cause of most disease is linked to toxicity. Dr. Becky tells us that 81% of our population is overweight and 18 million children in America are obese. Perhaps now you can see why it is vital to cleanse. In fact,

- You change the oil in your car.
- You brush your teeth.
- You clean the lint trap in your dryer.
- You change the bag in your vacuum regularly.

But do you cleanse your internal system on a regular basis?

Cleansing is the process of eliminating toxins from the body and detoxification is the natural process of filtering waste from the bloodstream, organs and cells. You have to flush those toxins out of your system to create ideal health. It is essential for lean people to cleanse because they have less fat to absorb the toxins, which go directly into their vital organs. Overweight people need to flush the toxins out along with excess body fat.

The Isagenix Nutritional System is your vehicle for better health, weight management and quality of life. This new food technology is the best available. It addresses cleansing, nutritional replacement and cravings through better nutrition. Everybody needs Isagenix.

Isagenix is not a fast or a diet, it is liquid nutrition. If you see a mother breastfeeding her baby, you would never say, "Why is that baby fasting?" Isagenix feeds the body all the vitamins and minerals it needs to provide the proper brain chemistry for optimum health and well-being.

Like parenting, the Isagenix Nutritional System is not something you pay attention to once and forget about. It is not a band-aid. It is a lifestyle—just like brushing your teeth or changing the oil in your car on a regular basis. Dr. Becky also says, "A little cleansing every day may keep the doctor away."

The Isagenix Cleanse for Life nutrient drink is a great tasting, herbal supplement that cleanses your liver. It contains a proprietary blend of trace minerals, inner-heart filet of aloe vera, organic herbal tea extracts and other specialized botanicals. The formula is designed to "feed" your body, not starve it, while you are cleansing—giving you a fast start to optimal health and weight loss.

Family Fitness

Another way you can inspire your family in a positive way is to follow the Surgeon General's warning which states that all children require exercise on a regular basis to fight obesity and other childhood diseases. You can influence your child's overall health and vitality by including physical activity in your daily routine. Get your children involved. Make sure that they see physical activity as fun instead of something they are required to do; don't force them to exercise. Begin with something your family can do together.

- Take a family walk after dinner.
- Turn off the television and go for a bike ride instead.
- Fly a kite together.
- Find a local ice rink and go ice-skating.
- Shoot hoops in the local park.

Respect your children's level of ability as you take time to discover which activities will appeal to them. Kids will continue exercising if they experience initial success, so start off slowly, keep it safe and be sure that they have fun. It is that initial success that will motivate your child to keep going.

In his book, *The Mars and Venus Diet and Exercise Solution*, Dr. John Gray says, "As your diet and exercise program help you sustain a high level of energy and well-being, making a relationship work stops being work." If your family relationships do not change overnight, don't give up. Change takes time and raising a family is a lifetime process.

When you and your family use the Isagenix products and receive the nutrients and amino acids your bodies require, you will find that you and your family will have more patience to effectively deal with school, work and stress. To help your body cope even better, take Isagenix™ Omega 3.6.9 gel caps daily. The high quality nutrients help support cardiovascular health, proper brain and neural development, good joint health and hormone balance.

Studies continue to link the lack of Omega-3 and 6 to the astounding rise of autism in children. Isagenix™ Omega 3.6.9 supplements may help your kids because they contain oils that are essential for brain function and development, which are lacking in modern processed diets. Omega-9 can also play a role in lowering cholesterol levels and promotes healthy inflammation responses. But not all fish oil and Omega-3 supplements are the same. Many supermarket and health food store brands are useless at delivering the essential fatty acids that your body needs. I recommend Isagenix™ Omega 3.6.9 for every body! They are convenient, easy-to-digest and do not have that "after fishy taste" or "burp reflex."

By taking good care of yourself, improving your communication skills and teaching yourself how to set an outstanding example for your family, you will give your children the gift of long-lasting health and happiness. At the beginning of each day, ask yourself what your kids would believe about themselves if their viewpoint were based solely on your words and actions. Then consciously send them positive, enriching messages. Create a safe, nurturing home environment in which your children can count on being heard, guided, respected and loved.

You are your child's best teacher; they learn how to communicate effectively from you. Practicing what you preach begins with a conscious decision to make a difference in your family's life. It is never too late to begin.

Take good care of yourself because I'm counting on you to take good care of your children.

Dr. Louise Hart

Keep Cool & Communicate

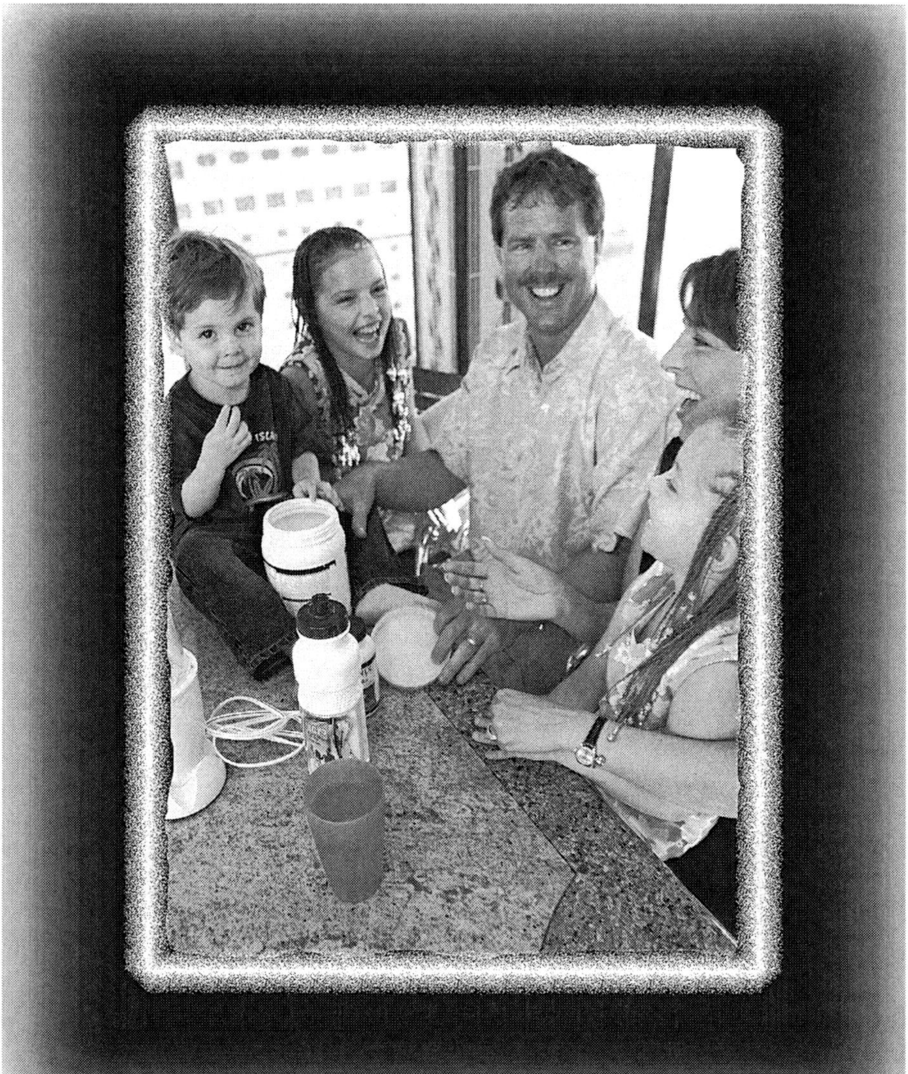

Chapter 4

Keep Cool & Communicate

Parents and children seldom speak the same language. Infants cry, toddlers speak gibberish and preadolescents talk incessantly. Teenagers, on the other hand, often slam their bedroom door and stop talking altogether. Frequently, they leave you standing alone and muttering to yourself out of sheer frustration.

No matter how hard you try to communicate effectively, at some point your children may throw tantrums and make you want to scream. If you rant and rave the situation will escalate and nothing will be solved—in fact, it could get worse. When your kids roll their eyes or turn their backs, your level of anger may continue to rise. By developing strong communication skills, you can remain calm and successfully get your point across.

When your children misbehave, give them an opportunity to learn from their mistakes without always giving a time-out or grounding them. Just sitting in a corner does not teach children how to respond to future dilemmas. Ask them how they could have handled the situation better. If your child responds with, "I don't know," then brainstorm solutions so they learn to think and problem solve on their own.

If you start to lose your temper, stop and take some time out for yourself. Before you walk away, calmly tell your kids, "I'm going to cool off right now. I will talk to you about this when I have thought about it some more. It's easier to talk when I'm calm instead of acting out in anger." Then leave the room before you say something you may regret later. If you do lose your cool, be forgiving with yourself and with your family. Apologize quickly if it is warranted, then start over again. This shows everyone around you how to take responsibility when they make mistakes. Behave in the manner you want your kids to emulate.

Children know that adults hold all the power. Your words, facial expressions, posture, tone of voice and attitude effect their basic belief about who they are and what they deserve in life. Much of what we reflect back to our children becomes the foundation for their self-image. This fundamental belief influences the choices they make and how they view every aspect of their lives.

Please keep these important points in mind when communicating with your kids:

- *Before you speak, think about what you say and how you say it.* Consider how you would react if someone spoke to you in the same manner. Remember, the words you use stay with your kids and affect their confidence and self-esteem.

- *Use teachable moments.* Find those moments in time when your children are willing to listen. You can often find a cooperative minute when you are driving in the car together or just before bedtime when everyone is calm and relaxed. Use this precious time to share your perspective or thoughtfully get a point across. If you lecture or preach, you may lose that teachable moment!

- *Listen carefully.* Acknowledge the importance of your kids' opinions when they express them. Wouldn't it feel great if someone actually gave you their undivided attention and put down the newspaper or turned off the television when you wanted to talk? Remind your children that their feelings and needs are important to you, and never tell them that their *feelings* are wrong. Be supportive, no matter how frivolous the issue may seem.

- *Speak to your kids with respect.* Don't interrupt when your kids are speaking; instead, show patience by listening to what they say. If you can't give them your undivided attention, let them know when you will be available—set up an appointment if you have to, instead of shrugging them off. By listening attentively, you show your kids that their concerns are important to you. Be polite, say "please" and "thank you" so family members learn to do the same. Don't belittle your kids. Speak in a tone of voice that is respectful and considerate, not demanding or harsh.

- *Apologize when appropriate.* Acknowledge when you are wrong or have made a mistake. Take responsibility for your actions. When your kids see that you are willing to admit to your mistakes and apologize, it makes you seem more real and sets a positive example for them.

- *Avoid criticizing or making judgments.* Kids often have a different perspective on life than adults. Sometimes they just want someone who will listen to their viewpoint without giving advice. If you have teenagers, ask if they want your opinion before offering it. We all know that kids don't listen when we lecture and saying, "I told you so" typically just pushes them away. Stay focused on what your children are trying to convey, even if it is difficult to follow. Listen with an open heart so they trust you enough to continue talking to you.

Set Boundaries

As children grow and learn about themselves, they need to know the guidelines and boundaries for their behavior. They will look to you for direction.

In my workshops, I encourage parents to set up their own family boundaries by drawing an imaginary box in their minds. That box contains your family rules, values and beliefs. The rules may differ slightly for everyone. Within this box, allow room for movement and flexibility so your kids can try on new clothes, new attitudes and different ways of being in the world. In other words, enable your kids to learn and grow in a safety zone within your own family boundaries. If your kids push out of that box by doing something illegal or dangerous, get a firm grip on the situation and reel them back in.

Setting fair boundaries and learning by thinking things through differs greatly from punitive punishment. Punishment usually inflicts mental or physical pain—which does not teach your child anything except to feel negative emotions and fear. Instead of blaming, grounding, threatening or bribing, think of yourself as a consultant instead of a manager. Work with your children to develop a game plan that works for the entire family. Everyone makes mistakes, but a true winner learns that success comes from trying, failing and persevering until you finally succeed.

Ask your kids what works for them. This gives them a sense of responsibility for their lives and provides them with decision-making opportunities. Seeking their advice can be a monumental step towards bridging the communication gap and teaching you both to speak the same language. However, family patterns are not transformed overnight; change takes awareness, skill and practice.

When you feel yourself becoming angry or impatient, be careful not to slip back into old, controlling or neglectful behavior. Keep calm and be understanding. Practice and trust your ability to communicate effectively. This will help you establish a more open, honest relationship with your family. Have faith in yourself and in your children.

> ***Children need love, especially when they do not deserve it.***
>
> *Harold S. Hulbert*

Include Love & Laughter in the Recipe

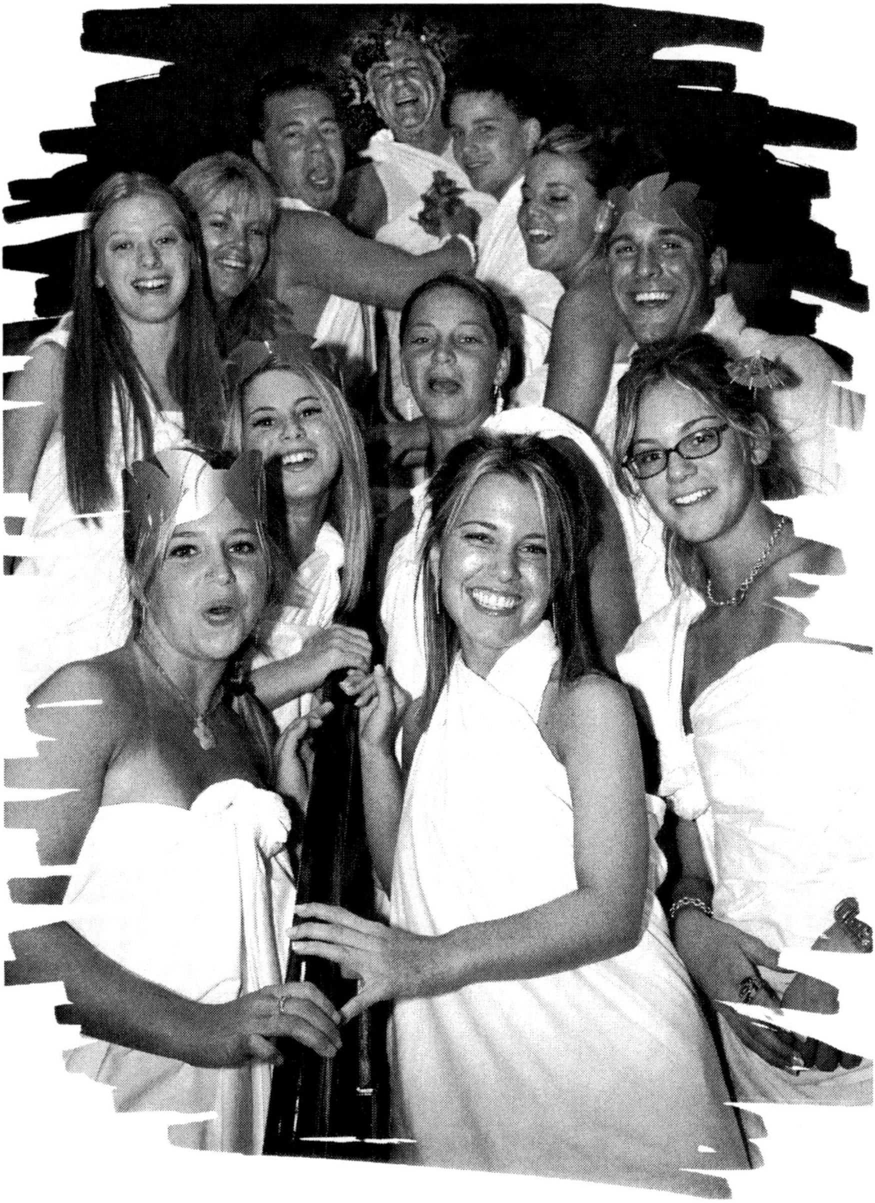

Chapter 5

Include Love & Laughter in the Recipe

Positive self-respect is a powerful force. It is the foundation for a well-adjusted and fulfilling life. Children who grow up feeling good about themselves are more secure and self-reliant. They function well in school and have greater trust in their own judgment.

Children need unconditional love in order to develop positive self-respect. Loving unconditionally means you love them for better or worse with no strings attached, even when they irritate you, defiantly challenge you or try to push all your buttons. You may be furious with their behavior, outraged by their attitude, or embarrassed by the way they dress. You do not have to approve of or like the situation, the behavior, or the attitude, but loving your children even when they act unlovable is the true test of unconditional love.

Some parents reserve their love and only express their appreciation when their kids please them: for example, when their children get good grades or do their chores. Positive reinforcement and kindness creates a special bond between you and your children so don't hold back. Create a warm, loving atmosphere and a place where your kids want to spend their time. Open your heart and joyously express your love, because each child is an absolute, unrepeatable miracle. If waves of love swept the world, waves of violence would not be possible. So don't just tell your kids that you love them, show them.

Guidelines to Live By:

1. Believe in your children, so they can believe in themselves.

2. Turn an accomplishment of any size into a celebration.

3. Praise your kids in public (but make sure not to embarrass them).

4. When your children talk to you, focus your attention on them and really listen.

5. Instead of saying "Hurry up and get to the point," be patient when they are talking.

6. Get down on the ground and play with your kids, even when they are big!

7. Give your little ones an appreciative smile or hug when they are gentle with animals.

8. When your kids get sick, give them extra love and attention.

9. Let both boys and girls know that crying is a natural human emotion.

10. Bestow sweet nicknames on them to use only in private.

11. Show how pleased you are when they are kind to younger kids.

12. Learn how to say, “I love you” in sign language and send “secret” messages to one another.

13. Notice your children’s bright ideas.

14. When your kids are home alone after school, call from work just to say, “I love you.”

15. Secretly wink at one another when you are in public, especially in a serious environment.

16. Thank them for showing respect to the elderly.

17. Take turns sharing a positive accomplishment every day.

18. If your kids are in the mood: sing, dance, and get really silly together—especially with your teenagers! (But don’t embarrass them).

19. Let them know how proud you are about the way they are growing up.

20. Take a class together.

21. Tell your kids what they have taught you.

22. When your children admit the truth about something they have done wrong, be sure to tell them how much you appreciate them for their honesty.

23. Make all consequences logical, reasonable and rational.

24. Teach your children to love by loving them and loving yourself.

25. Treat them as if this day were their last.

Everyone wants to be accepted and appreciated. When kids are young, parents express their love and praise freely. When they become adolescents, parents often forget to appreciate and praise them. Instead, they focus on their kids' mistakes. Show compassion when they make mistakes or let you down. Let them know that a mistake does not mean failure; it is a "miss take" and is a learning opportunity to try again.

Shower your kids with hugs, even when they are big; and remember how important it is not to embarrass them in front of their friends. If they don't want you to be openly affectionate, send silent kisses and invisible hugs when their friends aren't looking. You can't spoil a kid with too much love.

It has been said that laughter is the best medicine and can improve your child's health and behavior. A good laugh is a great aerobic workout for the heart and lungs. Laughter also increases the body's ability to use oxygen. According to a study from Duke University and UCLA, laughter can:

- Relax tense muscles.
- Help to lower high blood pressure.
- Reduce the production of stress hormones.

- Strengthen the immune system when combined with a positive attitude.

Repair your own sense of humor and boost your kid's energy level and mood by being playful and laughing. There are no known side effects to laughter and you are never too old or too mature to have fun. So do silly things like:

- Wear a clown nose when you tuck your kids in to bed at night.
- Have a spontaneous pillow fight in the middle of doing chores.
- Write your angry feelings on the bottom of your shoes and walk on them.
- Drink your Isagenix shakes together and "shake" while you drink.
- Dance around the room and tell jokes.

Share special moments such as bicycle rides, nature walks, cooking together or going to the movies to strengthen the bond between you and your child. Sing while you are doing dishes, prance around your kitchen and let yourself be goofy. Create an atmosphere in your home where everyone can be relaxed with one another. This is especially critical to maintain open communication with teenagers.

Don't turn every situation into a major issue. An unmade bed or messy room never killed anyone, so look beyond the less important things and don't take yourself so seriously. Being overly critical and negative takes so much effort. Your kids will be much more manageable if you aren't stressed out. Lighten up and keep problems in perspective. Children thrive in the tender loving care of a happy parent.

> ***I think the biggest disease this world suffers from in this day and age is the disease of people feeling unloved.***
>
> *Princess Diana*

Set Limits, Then Let Go

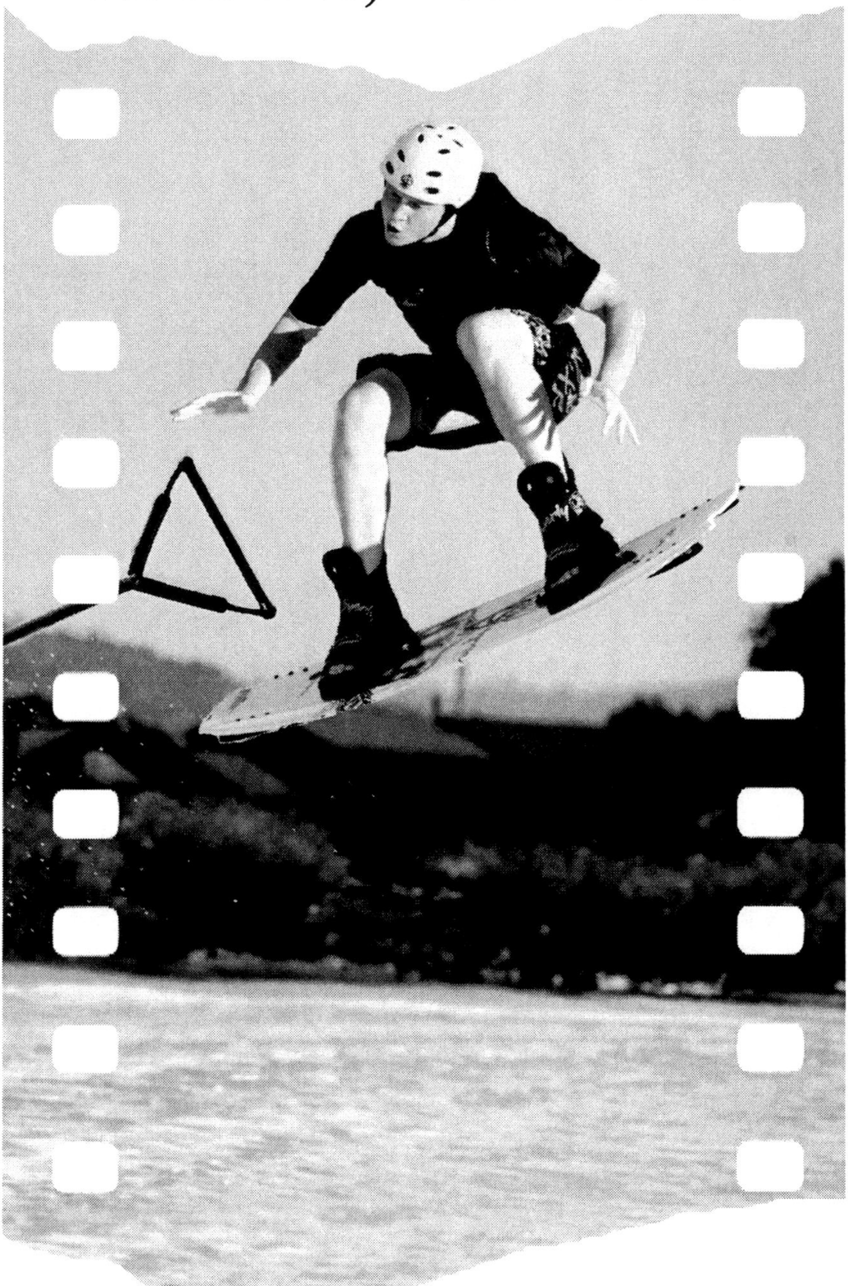

Chapter 6

Set Limits, Then Let Go

Separating from parents is a normal, natural process that begins when children utter their first, "No!" This separation and pushing-parents-away syndrome continues through adolescence and peaks during the teenage years. When this occurs, stop acting as your child's manager and become more of a guidance counselor. Parents who focus on remaining supportive and understanding instead of threatening and controlling, create a safe haven where kids can come with their unanswered questions and concerns.

The trick is to find a balance between holding on too tight and not being involved enough. Just because your teenagers have minds of their own does not mean they should be left to their own resources. Parents need to establish guidelines that inspire teens to use common sense and think things through.

When parents are too strict, kids end up with weak decision-making skills. When parents have weak boundaries and no clear-cut rules, kids often get out of control. When adolescents do not have the opportunity to constructively exert their power, they may take drugs, smoke, drink, become promiscuous, or over or under-eat to get back at their parents. These may be the only aspects of their lives they think they can control.

Therefore, it is imperative that you establish reasonable boundaries and rules within your home that each family member can live by. Ideally, this process begins when children are very young. Even though the boundaries change as kids mature, they still need to understand there are limits.

Allowing kids to participate in making up the family rules gives them an opportunity for active participation in their own lives. Teamwork and compromise will go a long way in bridging the gap that causes kids to rebel and over react. Work together with your children on a day-to-day basis to deal with issues your family may be able to compromise on, such as what they wear, chores, homework and curfew.

Remember to choose your battles. Is an unmade bed really worth the fight? Most teenagers' rooms are messy and their clothes pile up on the bedroom floor, but that does not really harm anyone. Set up clear boundaries and house rules by telling your kids to keep their bedroom door closed and keep the rest of the house clean. When they freak out because they can't find their favorite pair of jeans, calmly suggest they look for it in their room and let it become their responsibility, not yours.

An atmosphere of order without freedom sets kids up for rebellion, which may lead to lying and sneaking out. Save your strength for the things that really matter in your relationship with your child and what really matters in life.

When you set limits or say no to certain requests or behavior, expect anger, door-slamming and hard feelings. This is a normal reaction. Give your kids time to cool off and let them vent their disappointment and anger in their room. If your child gives you the cold shoulder, there is no reason for you to give it back. Be the example of strength and forgiveness.

Teens will make some unwise decisions, no matter what you do. The father of a fifteen-year-old boy told me, "If I picked my son up from a party and saw beer cans all over the place, I'd be really angry. I'd probably never let him go to a party again."

In such critical situations, let your child explain what was going on and listen to what he has to say. If you yank your kid out of the house and assume he is guilty, it tells him you can't trust him. If you react negatively without hearing his side of the story, he might come away from this situation thinking, "You don't trust me anyway, so I might as well drink." Kids need opportunities to learn to trust their own judgment and to prove to you that they are trustworthy.

In situations like this, it can take tremendous discipline and forethought not to fly into a rage. Instead of blowing up, say, "I want to take a few minutes to think about this," which goes over much better than, "I can't deal with your behavior. You're grounded!"

Whatever the issue may be, take time to cool off. When you resume the conversation, both you and your child will be more relaxed. Use these mistakes as teaching opportunities. Discuss what your child could have done differently and how situations like these can be avoided in the future. Take time to work things through with your kids so they can learn from the situation instead of feeling powerless, which often leads to more negative behavior.

Be There

Make yourself available as a sounding board. Remember you are a guidance counselor, not "the boss." Create an environment where your children feel it is safe to talk. Do this by really listening, respecting confidentiality and being supportive without judging. Some opening lines that often prove helpful when your older child is wrestling with a difficult situation include:

- I'm here to help you figure this out, if you want me to.
- I know you're upset about what's happening. Have you thought about some ways you might handle it?
- You've made good decisions in the past. I trust you'll make the best decisions in this case.

Of course there are exceptions to this approach. Where critical issues of health and safety are concerned, you must be assertive. For example, if your child is anorexic or bulimic, drinking and driving, practicing unsafe sex, or exhibiting violent behavior, then you have a responsibility to intervene. Get whatever help you need to deal with the problem. Talk to your doctor, minister or a school counselor. A family therapist can help mediate a conversation between you and your child when nothing you do seems to work. Short-term intervention may be all your family needs.

Everyone craves a sense of belonging and significance. I have been told by thousands of kids in my seminars that they feel left out and unimportant at home. Spend time together as a family. Include your kids in your Isagenix business and work toward a common goal. Give your children their own responsibilities. Make sure it is age appropriate, fun and something they can succeed at.

Get your younger kids to fold weekly newsletters. Older kids can call your success team and remind them of upcoming Isagenix conference calls. Teenagers can prospect by talking to their friends and teachers. Make Isagenix a part of your family and get your kids involved. Working together provides the extra bonus of spending quality time together. Include your kids in your life so they can learn how to create a healthy, happy life of their own.

Remember, the ultimate goal is to help your kids realize they are capable of making wise choices, so when they do leave home they can take care of themselves. Life happens. Hard times, heartbreaks, challenges and struggles provide them with opportunities rich with growth and potential knowledge. Letting go takes courage for both parents and kids. Use guidance, understanding, love and common sense—instead of depriving children of their dignity and respect—so they can grow up with a sense of autonomy as well as a connection to family, friends and society.

There are only two lasting bequests we can give our children. One is roots, the other is wings.

Hodding Carter

Schedule Time for Yourself

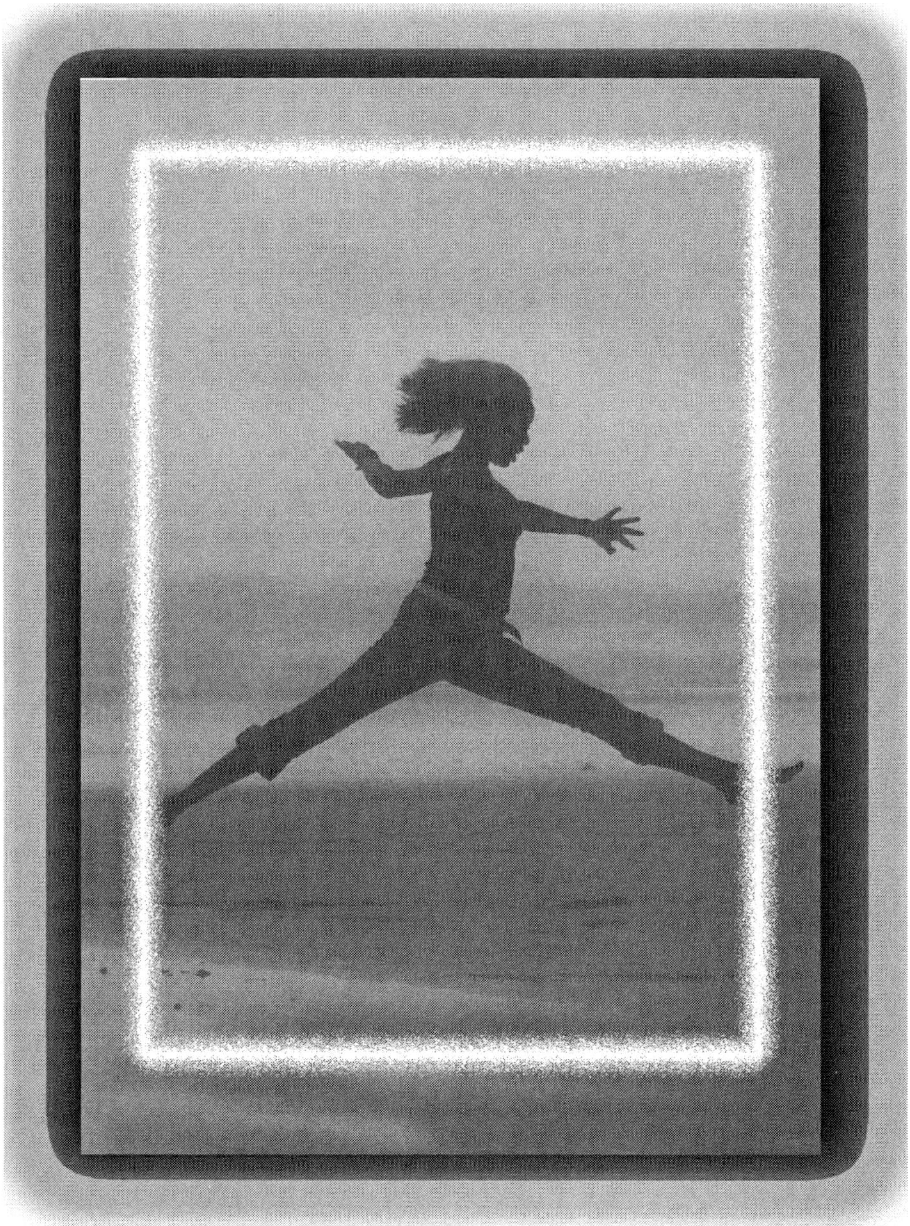

Chapter 7

Schedule Time for Yourself

Sometimes parents just need a break. When you are feeling overwhelmed, find ways to relax and gather your strength. Take a five-minute walk, a hot, soothing bath or just sneak away with a magazine and hide out so you can be alone. Do whatever you can to pamper yourself.

You may think you don't have time to indulge yourself, but there are ways of working down time into your busy schedule. When your baby is napping, lie down and relax. When your children are in school, visit your favorite bookstore, go shopping, get a massage, treat yourself to lunch or a movie, spend time in the garden or just listen to music. Take your mind off all the pressures and enjoy the pleasures of life.

If your kids are stressing you out, take a parenting class to learn new and more effective parenting skills. If your house is in disorder, clear up the clutter. Throw the laundry in a hamper, put the bills in monthly envelopes, clean up the kitchen and recycle those newspapers and magazines you never got to read. Everyone has his or her own method. Find out what works for you. You can also:

- Take tiny breaks throughout the day.
- If you have a desk job, change positions every 15 to 30 minutes; get up and stretch or walk around.
- Drink lots of water to keep your body adequately hydrated.
- Alternate tasks whenever possible to prevent boredom.
- Stand up to answer the phone.
- Climb the stairs instead of using the elevator.

By changing your actions and your thoughts you can transform your own reality. For example, taking frequent little breaks may not be a substitute for a week in Hawaii, but with a slight attitude shift you can create a most satisfying experience.

Switch a negative attitude to a positive one by focusing on the good things in your life. Live every day with full awareness, appreciation and gratitude. Focus on finding creative ways to feed your soul and nurture your body. Cherish every minute and make it count.

All your scheduling and prioritizing will not relieve your stress if you continue to do too much. If your family is stretched in every direction, something is bound to snap. Simplify your life. Create down time for yourself and your kids. Prioritize; save your time and energy for what matters most.

Clean Out Your Internal Closet

Many people believe that disease and stress are natural to the human condition. With all the turmoil and unrest in the world, there has never been a more urgent need for balance and purification. Negative thinking prevents us from experiencing our true potential.

Negative thoughts can get blocked in the body and disrupt our health. Purifying the body and keeping it supple will reduce the process of cell deterioration and can have a beneficial effect on numerous medical conditions.

Purifying is not limited to your internal organs. Stress, environmental toxins and overall health affect your skin as well. Men and women spend hundreds of dollars every month on skin care products so they can put their best face forward. Isagenix has created an affordable skin renewal system that is the most scientifically advanced renewal system in the world. Formulated by top scientists and plastic surgeons, The IsaDermix™ Skin Renewal System complements the Isagenix Health and Wellness System for internal and topical support of the skin. IsaDermix is recommended for all skin types and features:

- A leading-edge microdermabrasion technology. This proprietary process utilizes magnesium crystals and is 100% aluminum free.

- An advanced liposome system for fast, effective delivery.
- A revolutionary Vitamin C Collagen Serum formulation combining five forms of Vitamin C synergistically blended with collagen and other vital nutrients.

The IsaDermix Skin Renewal System also:

- Diminishes fine lines, wrinkles, rosacea, sunspots and acne.
- Revitalizes skin tissue to minimize stretch marks and scars.
- Refines the pores for smoother texture.
- Provides high protection against sunburn for you and your children.

With an all-natural approach, IsaDermix has been developed to make this anti-aging, skin rejuvenating treatment easier, safer and more convenient than other products on the market. The most exciting aspect of this cutting-edge technology is that every time you nurture your skin by purchasing IsaDermix, Isagenix International will donate a portion of sales to ChildHelp USA, an organization for the treatment and prevention of child abuse. You can nurture yourself and help a child in need at the same time. What a great way to start your day!

Stay Fit

In our ever-changing world with its frenetic pace of life, it is more important than ever to take care of your mind, body and spirit. Twenty years ago, I taught yoga and meditation worldwide. Yoga is a non-competitive, personal journey to greater health, mental control and ultimately, self-realization. The benefits of yoga can improve your overall physical health by increasing flexibility, toning your muscles and internal organs, increasing lung capacity, strengthening your bones and relieving inner tension.

To experience stillness and balance, wake up an hour earlier each morning and meditate. You can do it no matter how old or busy you are. There are many ways to meditate and even a few minutes on a daily basis can make a difference in the way you feel and think. Listen to the silence and feel the tension fade as you recharge your senses.

Don't forget to breathe. Breathe evenly through your nose to increase your relaxation. Inhale slowly for a count of five as you balloon your stomach outward. Then exhale slowly for a count of five and pull your stomach all the way in. When you gently and rhythmically balloon your stomach out, your diaphragm drops, which gives your lungs room to expand and take in more air. As you exhale and gently pull your stomach in, your diaphragm contracts and stale air is expelled from your lungs. By breathing properly your cells, tissues and organs maintain peak performance levels rather than becoming compromised and depleted.

To improve balance and coordination, try Pilates. The carefully designed exercises stretch and tone your body and increase strength and flexibility in your muscles and joints. You don't need fancy machines or hours in a gym; Pilates is a low-impact exercise that you can do at home.

There are many activities you can do at home to get yourself in shape. You can quickly transform your body from head to toe with the exercise tapes made for Isagenix by Gilad, the creator and star of America's #1 fitness show, Bodies In Motion. Gilad's aerobic workout sessions are easy to follow and a lot of fun. Get your kids to exercise with you as you all move to the music of the islands.

You and your kids will love the "Bounce and Shake" exercises in John Gray's Exercise video. John says, "The bounce and shake exercises, which are accompanied by some easy stretches from beginner's yoga, Pilates, Tai Chi, Chi Kung, and Callanetics, are all you need to activate your metabolism and stimulate brain chemistry." You and your kids will have more energy, increase oxygen supply to the brain and sleep better at night. Bounce and shake is easy to do and is great for older folks who do not have much flexibility or muscle strength.

If your energy drops during the day, Isagenix Want More Energy™ will reenergize you and safely get you going. It is a delicious and refreshing energy drink that comes in three flavors. It contains eighty-eight nutrients, is loaded with ionic and trace minerals and is one hundred percent drug and stimulant free. This natural electrolyte drink provides you with sustained energy and is great for pre and post workout. Instead of reaching for a candy bar, soft drink or those commercial, chemical-laden electrolyte drinks, try Isagenix Want More Energy at your kids' next soccer game or when you or your kids feel frazzled, tired or just need that afternoon energy boost.

Most of us don't associate what we ingest with stress or poor health, but what we eat has a direct impact on how we feel. Poor nutrition can cause moodiness, exhaustion, weakness and indigestion. As we already know, it can contribute to serious illnesses such as cancer, diabetes and obesity. Adjust your eating habits and modify your routine so you feel better and can cope with the ups and downs of everyday life.

IsaMune™, fondly known as the software for the human operating system, is nature's health enhancer. IsaMune contains the finest source of colostrum from cow's milk. We know that cow's milk provides our bodies with vitamin D and calcium, but our four-legged friends provide an even more powerful substance for our health: colostrum. Colostrum is the nutrient-rich, pre-milk fluid that is secreted by the mammary glands of female mammals to nourish their young. Bovine colostrum is nearly identical to human colostrum but research confirms it is four times richer in immune factors than human colostrum.

For those worried about lactose intolerance, worry no more! The small amount of lactose in IsaMune is less than that which has been shown to cause an allergic reaction in those sensitive to lactose. The proteins and proprietary technology in IsaMune insure maximum benefit and bioavailability. Children over the age of 3 years of age and adults can take 3 sprays twice daily. Infants and children under 3 years can use one spray twice daily.

If you feel a cold or flu coming on, then use IsaMune every 4 to 6 hours. Kids love the delicious vanilla taste.

Eating right and living a healthy lifestyle is only part of maintaining a healthy family. If your emotional nutrients are out of balance, nothing will work. The Isagenix system promotes the brain chemistry that ultimately affects your emotional state. When you are physically and emotionally depleted, you have nothing left to give. By incorporating Isagenix into your daily life, you can avoid running your tank on empty and focus on achieving peak performance.

The Rejuvenator

You can also count on Isagenix Ionix Supreme™. According to Isagenix founder and CEO, John Anderson, Ionix Supreme is a daily dietary supplement that is "The Spark Plug of Life." They also call it "The Destroyer of Weakness." This is by far the most comprehensive and ideal nutrient drink I have come across. Ionix Supreme contains Shilajit, which is a natural substance so pure and potent that it is perhaps the most nutrient-rich material on earth. Imagine a substance that is guaranteed to enhance your performance, support your health and increase your vitality. Fresh from the Humla Region high in the Himalayas of Nepal, Shilajit has been used for thousands of years. This powerful drink is Ph balanced and:

- Features Isalyte™, a proprietary blend of 70 ionic and trace minerals.
- Contains a Fulvic Acid delivery system which carries nutrients into the bloodstream.
- Helps to expel heavy metals from the body.
- Eliminates free radicals.
- Includes over 20 exotic herbal extracts such as Maca Extract, Wolfberry, Macuna and Bamboo.
- Helps balance and normalize body systems.

Proper nutrition is a part of each parent's health responsibility to their children and themselves. The Isagenix Nutritional System will help you to model healthy living habits. The rest is up to you. Stay positive and above all, let your children know they are loved no matter what.

Parenting, letting go and learning to trust take an incredible amount of courage. Creating good communication skills and healthy, strong, loving relationships takes time and effort. Consciously creating an environment of respect and reverence can be challenging. You don't need to be a super-parent to use the suggestions in this book. Simple respect, an understanding of the differences between adults and adolescents, a willingness to get along better and a lot of trust go a long way toward bridging the gap between parents and kids.

> ***You must be the change you wish to see in the world.***
>
> *Ghandi*

Listen to the Experts

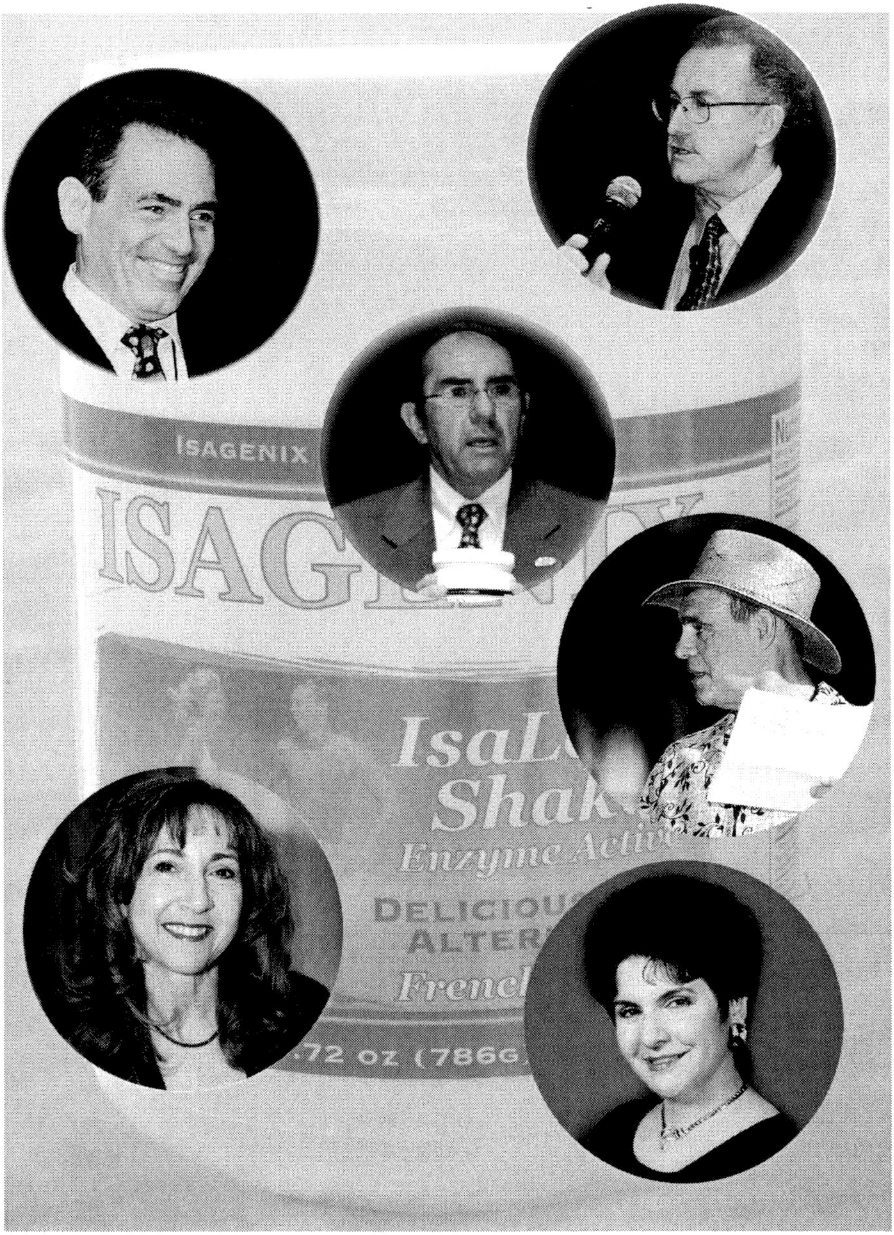

Chapter 8

Listen to the Experts

"It is wonderful to see an author who is interested in the health and welfare of children. Andrea has written a book that helps parents understand the necessity of good nutrition as well as positive parenting."

Dr. Dennis D Harper, D.O.
Medical Advisory Board
Isagenix International

Cynthia M. Watson, MD
Isagenix International
Medical Advisory Board

The largest resource that we have in the world is our children. How our children develop as human beings shape society and its values. How they are treated, loved and supported will shape the future of our world. As parents we have the opportunity to help them grow and become happy and balanced.

When we raise our children with self-esteem and self-worth, we give them a gift beyond any material possession. Children who feel good about themselves will make better decisions as adults. We have a responsibility to our children to treat them with respect, love and compassion. We have a responsibility to be the best role models that we can be.

Communication is the key. Children want to be heard and respected for their ideas. They count on us to provide them with appropriate limits. This goes for every thing, including what they eat.

Obesity and eating disorders are a major problem in our culture. Many of the current diseases such as arthritis, heart disease, and diabetes with all of its complications are linked to obesity. Research shows that high body fat creates an inflammatory process that accelerates disease. Even cancer is linked to diet and obesity. Women who are overweight have a much higher risk of developing breast cancer. Diets that are low in fiber, fruits and vegetables increase the risk of colon cancer. Many of these diseases could be prevented with a healthy lifestyle.

With high calorie-low nutrient food available to children at a low cost, the rate of childhood obesity is rising. We have created a society of unhealthy children who eat poorly and don't exercise.

Letting children eat junk food and empty calories without teaching them the importance of good nutrition is not only irresponsible, but also creates habits that may be difficult for them to break. Teaching them healthy habits when they are young will shape their lives forever. It is up to us as parents to establish awareness about good health.

With proper nutritional education, parental encouragement and understanding, we can teach our children the healthy habits they need to turn the tide towards a healthier future. The Isagenix Health and Wellness System provides the vitamins and nutrients that can help children achieve this goal.

George Boris
Certified Cosmetic Surgeon
Isagenix International Medical Advisory Board

My two-year-old daughter, Olympia, had a serious scar resulting from a burn. It became my mission to find an effective way to bring down my daughter's thickened, elevated scars. As a practicing Certified Cosmetic Surgeon in Beverly Hills, California for the last 34 years, I have used numerous techniques to eliminate skin problems including chemical peels, laser skin resurfacing and deep dermabrasion. I wanted to use something more natural for my little girl, without all the side effects the other treatments produced.

I began searching for a personal, easy-to-use microdermabrasion homecare system to enhance the other skin care products I developed. I wanted something that would eliminate the suction used in microdermabrasion that could cause disruption of the collagen elastic fibers or hematoma. I also wanted a system that would provide an advantage financially and time-wise over professionally administered treatments. The bottom line is, I wanted a safe program with natural botanicals that would work in harmony and could be used in the comfort of one's home.

As I developed the six-step Isagenix IsaDermix™ System, patients with chronic acne scars, stretch marks, cellulite and rosacea were finding great improvement. The microdermabrasion softened and developed new skin over my daughter's scar, making her able to deal with what could have been a serious disfigurement. We studied the changes microscopically and found new collagen and elastin had developed along with a healthier epidermis.

In the last decade, through a cosmetic fellowship program in my surgical center, I had many dermatologists, facial plastic surgeons, board certified plastic surgeons and chemists who helped create this skin renewal system. The system includes over 20 botanicals that reduce inflammation. It also includes special magnesium crystals that are natural and have a very controlled action that make it extremely effective on very sensitive skin.

The products have many antioxidants including Superoxide Dismutase (SOD), the world's strongest antioxidant, along with many vitamins. This system utilizes the most advanced liposomal delivery system to provide ultra deep penetration of nutrients and vitamins into the skin.

The Vitamin C Serum in the IsaDermix System is a composite of five different types of vitamin C. Each bottle of our serum contains 10% of the finest Vitamin C available in the world. Vitamin C extends into the deeper levels of skin to seek out and bind to potentially dangerous molecules.

In essence, we have formulated a six-step system with the mildest ingredients possible, including Noni Fruit Juice, Arnica, Comfrey, Kelp, Cucumber, Green Tea, Marshmallow, Red Clove, White Lily Extracts, Tangerine Oil, Kava Kava Root and many other components to protect the skin.

IsaDermix is revolutionary. The quality of ingredients is sourced from around the world and they are outstanding. The products work in harmony with each other to cleanse, replenish and revitalize the skin. We use aluminum free magnesium oxide crystals in the skin revitalizing treatment, which is simply not known to the conventional cosmetic and dermatology community. IsaDermix is the most scientifically advanced skin renewal treatment available anywhere in the world today. All my patients love it and the beauty of the system is, not only does it work, but people are continually using it and reordering it.

The Isagenix Nutritional Program cleanses the inside of your body and the IsaDermix Skin Renewal System cleanses the outside. Together, they create a complete program for overall health and well-being. Coupled with Andrea's indispensable tools for sound nutrition, effective family communication and understanding, I believe we have a home remedy for the problems of human suffering. Thank you Andrea. Way to go Isagenix!

Thomas McNeilis, M.S., D.O., F.A.C.O.G., Nutritionist Isagenix International Medical Advisory Board

As a nation, we are faced with a very difficult crisis—that of obesity at epidemic proportions. Of particular concern are the children. More than one in five young Americans are overweight or obese. Many of them will become overweight adults, putting these individuals at risk for stroke, hypertension, diabetes and other chronic diseases.

Young people today have become less physically active in their daily lives and tend to pursue more sedentary recreation; over 25% watch television at least four hours per day. Instead of snacking on fruits and vegetables, children tend to eat more fast food saturated with fat, which contributes to obesity.

We can no longer sit back and watch this epidemic continue. Every child deserves a healthy start and nutrition is critical. Parents need to be ready and willing to be responsible for their children's nutrition and healthy lifestyle.

Skipping breakfast may be part of the problem. A good morning meal is one of the most important contributions you can make to academic success, providing that meal includes nutritious food. Eating a nourishing breakfast can improve academic performance, enhance working memory, increase verbal skills and improve math scores. Studies also show that kids have improved attitudes toward school, as well as less depression, anxiety and hyperactivity.

Trying to decide what to fix that is nutritious, fast and easy can become a problem, especially if your kids aren't hungry or you are rushing out the door. The nutritious IsaKids shake contains all the protein, vitamins, essential amino acids, trace minerals and enzyme transport systems needed to give the brain and body everything it needs.

In my practice, parents report positive and significant changes in their children's behavior when IsaKids is instituted in the home. Good health begins with parents who pass along healthy values and eating habits to their children. Isagenix is a great start towards decreasing the obesity epidemic in adolescents.

Tony Escobar
Isagenix Advisory Board Member

The IsaKids formula represents a unique meal in the form of a delicious smoothie, rich in immune supporting whey protein. This is not your ordinary whey; the amino acids are not added, they occur naturally. The 70-plus trace minerals which every child needs, are harvested from ancient plant beds millions of years old.

IsaKids is loaded with vitamins especially folic acid, B-12, biotin and minerals as well as specially selected botanicals and honey. Many children today are constipated due to the extensive ingestion of processed foods; the IsaKids smoothie is rich in special fibers that promote regularity.

Perhaps the best aspect of all is that IsaKids has no added white sugar. It is a rich, wholesome food that supports the immune system and promotes beautiful, healthy skin and hair as well as mental clarity.

There is not a child in America that cannot benefit from this evolutionary formula. Yes indeed, evolutionary, as it evolved from the deficiencies associated with those other protein meal replacement drinks on the market. The IsaKids Super Shake represents wonderful, beneficial nutrition that promotes good health and an active lifestyle. On a personal level I cannot think of a finer product to give my grandchildren.

Marilyn Territo, C.E., C.M.
Clinical Skin Fitness Expert
Author of
Ionix Supreme: The Rejuvenator

Good nutrition is an important part of an anti-aging program, and it is essential to skin health. The Isagenix Health and Wellness System is easy to incorporate into anyone's lifestyle. It provides the vital nutrients required by the body daily to maintain a high-level of wellness and skin fitness.

The acclaimed Ionix Supreme is part of the Isagenix program. Ionix is a nutrient-dense supplement drink that contains 29 proven ingredients sourced globally from Mother Nature's healing garden. There are over 100 bio-active agents in these botanicals, including a proprietary blend of 70 organic minerals and ionic trace minerals. Nine of these ancient and exotic herbal extracts are powerful anti-stress adaptogens. Botanicals and vitamins, rich in free-radical fighting antioxidants, add to the rejuvenation benefits of this supplement drink.

While there are many valuable ingredients that support sexual health in Ionix, there are seven that are especially noteworthy for sexual well-being for both men and women: Maca Root, Siberian Ginseng, Schizandra, Ginger Root, Velvet Bean, Ashwaghanda, and Shilajit. As with all the quality ingredients selected for Ionix, the water is no exception. Isagenix uses ancient water that has pooled and flowed in the largest quartz crystal mine in the world located in the state of Arkansas. The water contains high concentrations of oxygen, minerals, and trace minerals which are miniscule power nutrients. Ionix Supreme is incomparable for its restorative benefits for body and skin enhancement. As a natural supplement blend, it supports you in reclaiming passion in all areas of your life. This is why this energizing drink has popularly become known as The Rejuvenator!

IsaDermix™ is the most advanced skin renewal system currently available on the market. It is the blending of leading-edge skin science and technology, medical-esthetics, and the art of skin care. The six unique products in this system were formulated and clinically tested and proven to provide maximum benefits for the skin of the face and body. The system can be used by both men and women for skin health and diminishing of the visible signs of aging. When used daily, morning and evening, the program will repair, rejuvenate, and protect the skin. It is a rare opportunity for consumers to be able to purchase and use medical-esthetics/spa grade skin care products in the privacy of their homes.

When you combine the Isagenix nutritional products with the IsaDermix Skin Renewal System, you have the most leading-edge and comprehensive wellness program available today for healthy-aging and longevity. I personally use both the Isagenix Nutritional System and the IsaDermix™ Skin Renewal System, and I highly recommend it to my clients, audiences, and readers!

Testimonials

It gives me such peace of mind to know that my children are getting the very best in nutritional supplements with Isagenix. They love the IsaLean Shakes and most of all, they love the Slim Cakes! My husband and I will never go a day without it. It has helped us slim down and feel more energy than ever before. I'm so thankful for Isagenix, and for my awesome dad, John Anderson, I love you! Thank you for helping our little family and the entire Isagenix Family regain health, strength and vitality. I feel very privileged to be a part of something so grand.

Kjersti Cote
Kalispell, Montana

The Isagenix program for children takes the stress out of nutrition for parents and kids. We have a group of happy, healthy families with Isagenix and what better can we do for people.

Kathy Coover
Co-founder Isagenix

I am an athlete and an avid surfer. I like the Isagenix program because it gives me extra stamina and the energy to play longer and better. It's easy to use and tastes great.

Jace Dispenza, age 15
Malibu, CA

My husband and I have been in the nutritional food arena for over 20 years. We have never before seen a product like IsaKids. I wish it had been around when I was raising my 4 children. I am thankful that it exists today so I can share it with my grandchildren. The children love the taste of their Cookies and Cream shakes which gives them a source of great nutrition to start their day off right. The kids also use it as an after school snack to replenish their system, help them concentrate on their homework and participate in their sports programs. We love that they love IsaKids!

Randi Escobar
Salt Lake City, UT

I like the flavor of the snacks. I like to suck on 'em. I can make 'em last a long time and the chocolate one tastes like a tootsie roll!

Spencer Ganus, age 5
Toluca Lake, CA

Every morning before school, our three daughters, ages 4, 6 and 9, have their Ionix Supreme. Then we spray the IsaMune into all three waiting mouths. This saves us a lot of time and money because they do not catch colds like they did before. Our girls are healthier now that their immune systems are in optimal condition thanks to Isagenix. We also give our kids the best of the best snacks at school. They each get an IsaLean Chocolate Bar and a frozen, Want More Energy Drink every day. Isagenix is a blessing because it has made our Puerto Rican family happier and healthier.

Kerensa Luciano and Roberto Pérez
Toa Alta, Puerto Rico

We started out by giving our three-month-old daughter an ounce of Fast Start with water followed by some IsaLean shake in her goat's milk. Marissa is now 17 months old and loves her Isagenix shakes. I know that she is getting great nutrition with the Isagenix products.

Kim Kelley and Ray Ewing
Napa, CA

Both our children are living proof that love, Cool Communication and proper nutrition produce miraculous, kind, loving individuals. There is "No-Thing" more important than a happy home! We must first be the change we want to see. Be the example as best you can. It starts at home, with YOU!

Beth Miller
Isagenix Advisory Board
Malibu, CA

This past spring, we introduced the IsaLean shakes to our two small children. They love them! The shakes soon became a part of our morning ritual with both children sipping them on the 15-minute drive to school. We are grateful that Isagenix cares enough about the nutritional needs of children to develop such incredible products.

John & Janet Burton
Phoenix, AZ

I asked my two year old if she likes her daily Isagenix shake. Sophia simply said, "Yuumm!"

Cynda Williams
Los Angeles, CA

I'm 15 years old and I used to weigh 325 pounds. I lost 15 pounds and 5 inches around my waist in my first week on Isagenix. I've lost a total of 125 pounds in 10 months. Before I lost all that weight I was depressed and snapped at everyone. The first thing I noticed when I started the Isagenix program was that my attitude changed dramatically. I went from being depressed to feeling happy, calmer and thinking about what I wanted to say. I have more energy and can do things I couldn't do before.

Jarrett Christiansen
Tucson, AZ

I love the Isagenix shakes because my cravings for junk food and sugar are gone. If I get hungry during class, I pop a Snack in my mouth when no one is looking, which makes me feel a lot better. I'm not the best cook, so when no one is home, I just whiz up a shake and I feel completely satisfied. I love all the Isagenix products!

Gianna Dispenza, age 14
Malibu, CA

Isagenix is the most amazing gift our family has ever received. It has been one of those golden opportunities that have afforded us the ability to touch countless numbers of people's lives and fill them with the abundance of health, wealth and happiness. Isagenix is the vehicle that has taken us to the place where all of our dreams and desires are coming true!

Laurie and Kelly Moore
Pleasant View, UT

Spencer is a notoriously slow eater, but the minute we set a shake in front of her, it disappears in moments. Sometimes we add yogurt, ice cream or frozen fruit. It's nice to know she's getting 17 grams of protein, especially since she doesn't eat red meat. When my kids ask for candy or treats, I give them Isagenix Snacks, which is much healthier for them. Sometimes the kids put together little "tea parties" and fill their teacups with the Cookies and Cream IsaKids shake. Between the shakes and the snacks, their blood sugar stays stabilized for quite a while. Needless to say, that makes for more enjoyable play dates for everyone.

Ellen Bradley and Paul Ganus
Toluca Lake, CA

I am a stay-at-home mom with three boys under the age of seven. I am passionate about what these products can do. As I share Isagenix with family and friends, my kids learn the importance of helping others. My children have a delicious IsaLean shake each morning and they help me with my Isagenix business. Braxton, my 5-year-old, loves to put labels on my brochures and flyers. Stockton, 7, loves to staple and add stamps to my envelopes. 3-year-old Walker sits on my lap while I am online or working on the team newsletter! I love how Isagenix has brought my family together and continues to do the same for families everywhere.

Kimber King
Riverdale, UT

Isagenix is pure nutrition for children. It provides them with the brain chemistry they need for acceptable behavior and exceptional learning.

Jana Ridenour
San Jose, CA

Isagenix has been the best health decision I've ever made for my family. Our 17-year-old had extra pounds to lose and did the 9-day cycle during finals. She was more alert and clear thinking than usual and felt great! Our slender 8-year-old starts the day with breakfast and a shake. She loves the taste and I feel better knowing she's getting the nourishment she needs. We use the products consistently because we feel a greater sense of calm, patience and well-being. The whole family works and plays better. Thank you, John Anderson, and thanks to my dear friends who introduced me to Isagenix.

Becky Geist
San Rafael, CA

Life-long exercise fanatic Dana couldn't lose the last 7 pounds to get into a special dress for a family event. Larry, once an Atkins devotee gained his weight back and 12 year-old Matt had headache problems. Then came Isagenix. Dana now fits into her 1988 wedding dress, Larry lost 30 pounds and has enormous energy and Matt feels better than ever from the amino acids in the IsaLean shake.

Larry and Dana Weinberg
Los Angeles, CA

It's amazing how parent's behaviors and habits rub off on their children! After 18 months of enjoying the Isagenix Nutritional System, my 2_ year old son lead me to the pantry for his afternoon treat. Not fully understanding everything he was saying, I went through a process of elimination as I picked up packages of cookies, crackers and cereal. When he finally said, "Genix Snack," I reached for the bottle of Vanilla Snacks. My son smiled and nodded, "yes!" What a great feeling to know his little body actually wanted something balanced and nutritious! Because good nutrition is so important for kids, especially first thing in the morning, we no longer have bowls of cereal for breakfast. Instead, my family of five all enjoys a healthy shake together. We start our day the right way! Thanks Isagenix!

Kathy Humpherys
Draper, Utah

Healthy Family Recipes

Smoothies and slushies made with the IsaKids or IsaLean shakes make colorful, fruit-filled treats prior to a sports game or for an afternoon pick-me-up. The protein in the shake will provide energy while managing your children's appetite. Let your kids invent new recipes and have fun!

If you and your kids create a recipe that you would like to share with the entire Isagenix Family, please email it to me at andrea@coolcommunication.com.

The Moore Pleasant Smoothie

4 ounces 100% Apple Juice (no sugar added)
2 ounces Tropical Cleanse for Life Drink
½ banana and 2 or 3 strawberries
Lots of ice cubes
Blend in the IsaBlender (safe for kids)
Slurp Away!

The Moore Kids
Shae, Aubrie and Teagan
Pleasant View, UT

Blueberry Bliss

2 scoops Vanilla IsaLean Shake
8 ounces cold water
1 handful of fresh blueberries
Add ice and blend

The Dispenza Kids
Jace and Gianna
Malibu, CA

School Substitute

1 packet Chocolate or Vanilla IsaLean Shake
8 ounces water
Manual travel blender
Add ingredients and shake until blended

Nikki Dizon
Yelm, WA

Tropical Treat

2 scoops Vanilla IsaLean Shake
8 ounces cold water
Sliced fresh or frozen papaya, mango and pineapple
Small scoop of coconut sorbet
Add ice and blend

The Henkart Kids
Journey and Quest
Marin County, CA

Chocolate Decadence
2 scoops Cookies and Cream IsaKids Shake
½ banana
Small serving mint chocolate chip ice cream
8 ounces cold water
Blend in IsaBlender

The Ganus Kids
Spencer and Tyler
Toluca Lake, CA

Cherry Delight
2 scoops Chocolate IsaLean Shake
8 ounces cold water
½ banana
½ cup frozen cherries
Add ice
Blend for 10 seconds in the IsaBlender

The Reid Kids
Aria and Paris
Yelm, WA

Ice Cream Imposter
Blend 8 ounces of water and lots of ice to create ice cream-like thickness
Add 2 scoops Cookies and Cream IsaKids Shake
Quickly blend for 1-2 seconds to keep cookie pieces intact
Eat with a spoon!

Nick Gibson
Yelm, WA

Berry, Berry Yummy

2 capfuls of Berry Cleanse for Life
2 scoops chocolate shake
Handful of ice
Blend in IsaBlender

Jerilee Geist
San Rafael, CA

Texas Tea

1 ounce of Ionix Supreme
12 ounces purified water
Juice from 2 organic lemons
A pinch of Stevia
Add ice and stir
Grab a straw and sip away!

The Kelly Kids
Eliza, Elliot, Anna and Sam
Keller, TX

California Cooler

2 scoops of Vanilla IsaLean Shake
8 ounces of water
8 ice cubes (ice dispenser size)
2 scoops Vanilla Bean Haagen-Dazs Ice Cream
1 medium to large banana
Mix well in IsaBlender

The Macker Kids
Miranda, James and Joe
San Diego, CA

Dressing & Dipping

Mix together and refrigerate:

1 cup organic non-fat yogurt
1 tsp. fresh dill (chopped fine)
1 tsp. sun-dried tomato (chopped)
½ tsp. curry powder
1 clove garlic (minced)—optional

In a separate bowl, add 2 scoops Isagenix Creamy Chicken Soup to 3 ounces of hot water (not boiling)

Just before serving, mix water and soup mix together and stir well

Combine with the yogurt mixture

Use as a creamy salad dressing or dip for raw veggies

Consume within 20 minutes

1/4 cup = 1/4 meal replacement

The Anderson Kids
Jared, Austin, Nicholas, Cody, Savannah & Shelbie
Sacramento, CA

Puerto Rican Pasta

Prepare enough pasta for the entire family
Set aside
Stir enough IsaLean Creamy Chicken Soup into a small amount of hot water to create a sauce-like thickness
When thick, pour over pasta
¡Buen Provecho!

The Perez Kids
Kereisha, Diane and Monik
Toa Alta, Puerto Rico

About the Author

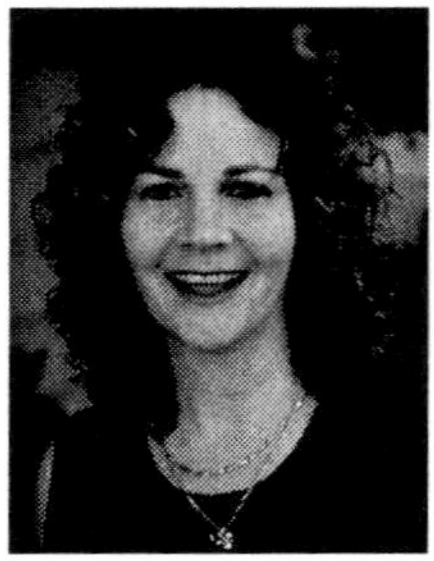

Andrea Frank Henkart is an internationally recognized expert and popular keynote speaker specializing in the fields of parenting, communication skills and personal development. She has two teaching credentials from UCLA and a Master's Degree in Psychology.

From 1978-1985, Andrea received numerous degrees and certifications in various health oriented philosophies including Holistic Health, Massage Therapy, Natural Childbirth Assistant and Yoga.

Also known as the Babysitter Expert, Andrea teaches a unique blend of professionalism, safety skills and leadership in her popular workshop *Super Sitters: A Positive Approach to Babysitting*. She has personally taught over 10,000 preteens and teenagers nationwide.

Andrea is the author of three books: *The Cesarean Challenge (1991)*, *Trust Your*

Body! Trust Your Baby! (1995), *and Cool Communication: From Conflict To Cooperation for Parents and Kids (1998)*, which she co-wrote with her daughter, Journey, who was 15 years old at the time. Journey currently holds a BA in Sociology from UCSB.

Both Andrea and Journey serve on the Board of Directors for Parents and Teachers Against Violence in Education. They are frequent guests on radio and TV and have been featured on Oprah Winfrey and Montel Williams.

Companies, associations, schools and individuals around the world have benefited from Andrea's keynote presentations, seminars and workshops. Her success strategies have inspired thousands of people of all ages to develop effective communication skills to reduce conflict in families, communities and the workplace.

Please call Andrea's office at 415-382-7755 for booking information, or visit her website at www.coolcommunication.com to learn more about her seminars for your family or business.

About the Photographer

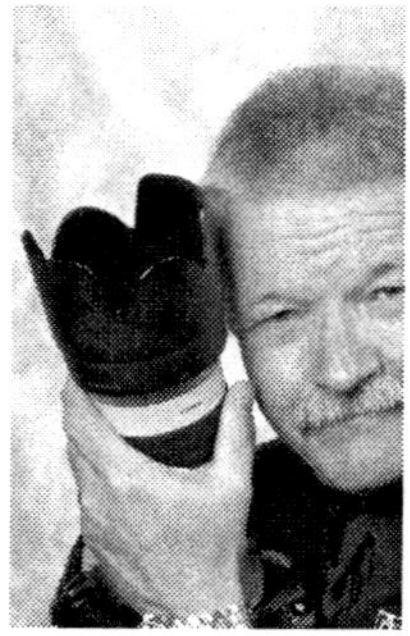

Reggie Henkart, an award-winning photographer from Belgium, has been capturing the essence of personality and feelings since 1969.

He has worked with major corporations such as Club Med, MCI, Great Expectations, The Mars Venus Institute and Isagenix International. Reggie has photographed numerous celebrities, many of which can be seen in his book, *100 Faces of Marin* (www.100faces.org), 2004. He is a member of Professional Photographers of America, Wedding and Portrait Photographers International and the National Association of Photoshop Professionals.

Using a photojournalistic approach, Reggie captures the heart of weddings in castles, wineries and on yachts internationally. His repertoire also includes the acclaimed, *A Day in the Life of your Family;* a personalized coffee table book filled with precious images of the family. Contact Reggie at reggie@limage.net.

Parenting & Motivational Resources

Books:

The Healthy Family Handbook: Creating Physical & Emotional Nutrition at Home $14.95

Cool Communication: From Conflict to Cooperation for Parents and Kids $15.95

Trust Your Body! Trust Your Baby! $14.95

Audios/CDs:

Building Winning Relationships at Work and at Home: Live at the Million Dollar Round Table
PLUS
The Healthy Family Handbook: an Interview with Andrea for Isagenix International
2 CDs for the price of 1! $14.95

Recordings from Andrea and Journey's radio interviews, teleconferences, stage presentations and workshops available upon request.

To order, please go to www.coolcommunication.com.

Create Health & Harmony at Home!

Share this book with your Isagenix Team Members.

The Healthy Family Handbook................$14.95

10-pack..$99.00

100-pack...$795.00

(plus applicable sales tax, shipping and handling)

—All prices subject to change without notice—

For more information, please contact: